Sit In Yo Sh*t:
A 30-Day Guided Journal for Processing a Crisis

Devin Elisse

COPYRIGHT

Sit In Yo Sh*t
'A 30-Day Guided Journal for Processing a Crisis'
Copyright © 2023 by **Angela Marie Publishing, LLC**

Original manuscript written by
Certified Life Coach & Founder of Lifted KC, Devin Elisse

Published for print under **EMEYEU Literature & Truth's Haven**
from **Angela Marie Publishing, LLC**

Angela Marie Publishing
4220 Duncan Ave
Suite 201-AMP
St. Louis, MO 63110
www.angelamariepublishing.com

ISBN: 978-1-954981-00-3 (PRINT EDITION)

DEDICATION

I dedicate this book to any person that has ever questioned God or asked, "why me?"!!

Just because things look like they were sent to destroy you, doesn't mean that is God's intent. I challenge you to thank God for allowing difficult experiences to happen to you!

Genesis 50:20, NLT version
"You intended to harm me, but God intended it all for good. He brought me to this position so I could save the lives of many people."

For a long time, I considered myself a victim! Even in the cases where I literally *was* the victim, I didn't let that title consume or keep me in a place of pain. I discovered that there is an outlet – *healing*! It wasn't until I began to HEAL that I realized God was using ME to help and inspire others to HEAL!

It's hard being vulnerable because sharing your story means welcoming opinions, criticisms, and even hatred into your world. BUT it also means inspiring, encouraging, uplifting, and giving a voice to those who may not be as bold. Those latter reasons are far more worthy than the negative implications of the former!

I'm honored to be a spokesperson for US; a light to the dark; a hope!

Lastly, I also dedicate this journal to my children – DreVeyon, Alonni and Ariq – whose lives awakened mine. I'll forever live for you 3 because you all are MY INSPIRATION!

- *Devin Elisse*

Table of Contents

Preface...xi
Foreword...xvii
Childhood Trauma.....................................21
The Situation...49
The Man in the Mirror...............................73
My Supporters...111
The Come-up..143

cri·sis (ˈkrī-səs):

"a time of intense difficulty, trouble, or danger that leaves you with more questions than answers."

Similar to crisis:

trauma, catastrophe, setback, adversity, drama

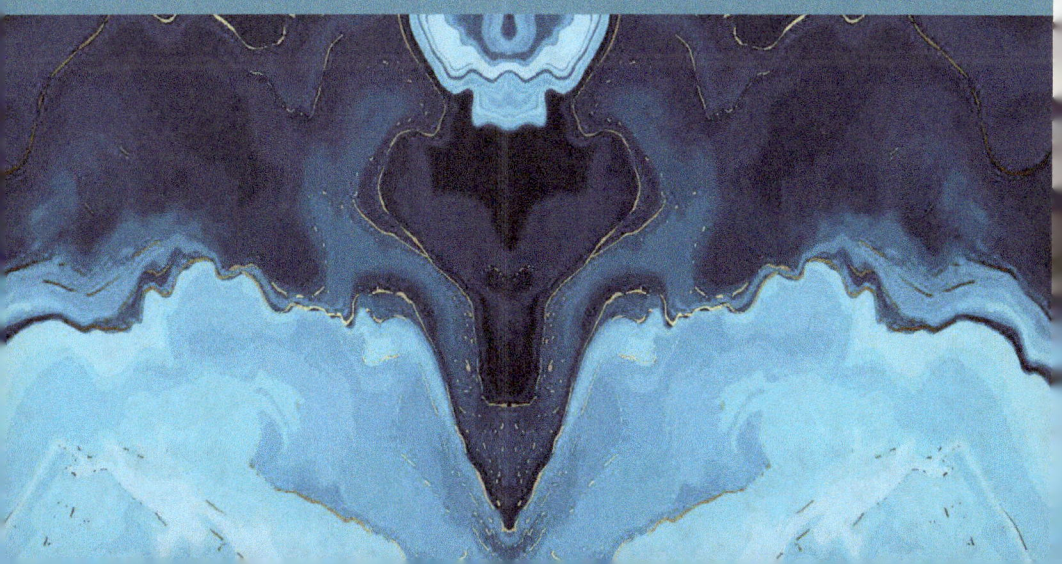

PREFACE

A Word from the Author

This book will consist of short snippets of my personal story. My experience with my second husband put me on my ass – literally! I was completely blindsided and caught off guard by what happened. You'd think that having been divorced once before, I'd kinda be knowledgeable on a wounded marriage – but this one hit different. And it hit HARD. Fortunately, I was all alone and had time to really process the events that transpired and later was able to look back on things that led up to the day.

Learning how to *sit in yo shit* will create an opportunity for you to analyze the things that got you to the point of needing to heal. Your story or situation may not be the same as mine. Whether your situation is a wounded marriage, divorce, failed relationship or friendship doesn't matter! It could even be the inability to have a healthy co-parenting relationship, losing a job, grieving the loss of a loved one, or a disagreement with family! We know the discussions can be endless in any of these scenarios, however, the outcome should be common: *to heal from the trauma/pain caused.*

Sometimes we all need to just take a minute to sit back As a culture – we've created the desire to push through, push forward, and keep it moving…with no consideration to resolution or healing. I'm not saying that moving on is a bad thing, but to move forward and NOT heal can be very detrimental to your future. On the contrary, healing while moving forward in a healthy manner comes with a lot of self-reflection, accountability, encouragement for changed behavior and forgiveness. All of these steps are necessary to healing!

This journal is a 30-day journey where you'll be challenged to take an honest look at your raw self and acknowledge things that will hopefully create a desire for changed behavior. Whether your experience is past or present, use this time to literally *sit* in the pain, reflect on the pain, and start the healing process. Do not expect to be perfect in this journey. Do not expect to complete this process in 30 days exactly. Be gentle and patient with yourself. Allow for downtime in which you do nothing. There may be days when you don't even open this book! But for your sake – make sure you come back and *keep* coming back until you reach the finish line . Healing is a marathon – not a sprint! There's no set timeframe on how long it should take; just be intentional every day to walk the journey.

Remember, healing is a daily process and requires you to be honest with YOURSELF!

Healing is also an intentional action that requires doing the work, sitting in our pain, analyzing how we can do things differently in the future, and applying those newfound changes. Most of the time we are quick to focus on the negatives, which then causes us to miss the insight of the positives. So instead of saying *'hurt people hurt people'*, let's strive to become a community of people who instead emphasize:

Healed people, heal people.

It is my prayer that you trust the process. Our situations will not be identical; our pains and feelings may not coincide. But trust that some of the mistakes I've made can indeed prevent you from making the same mistakes. I pray that you take each day seriously and really use this guide to process through your healing journey.

This is not the beginning! I'm not promising you eternal healing (if that's even a thing)! But I am offering you a chance to veer down a path of something that could be life altering! Will it be hard? HELL yes! Will it hurt? ABSOULETLY! Will it be draining? Some days, yes. But trust me when I say, it's REWARDING! When you get through that darkness and finally start to see the light – boy, does that light shine bright!! That light will provide a clearer vision, a place of joy, and an opportunity to live life with peace!

While going through this journal, I ask that you try to focus on *one situation*. Keep in mind that you can apply this guide to several situations over and over – but try not to overwhelm yourself and deal with one thing at a time…if you can help it. I encourage you to order a different journal for each situation you'd like to process and keep them all! 😊

Finally, be committed! No matter what – commit to writing on subject or answer the question of the day. Complete your assignments! I don't care if this 30-day process turns into 60 or 90 days – just complete it. Again, healing can be painful. So I urge you to take all the necessary emotional breaks and seek support from close family members or friends. Still reach out to your therapist, life coach, and/or other mental health professionals – but don't stop until you get to the last page! I promise it'll be as rewarding as it sounds and there's a gift for you at the end – figuratively and literally speaking!

Join me on my journey and know that I am also walking with you through yours!

Stay the course! I wish you peace, love, and blessings on your healing journey.

- Devin Elisse

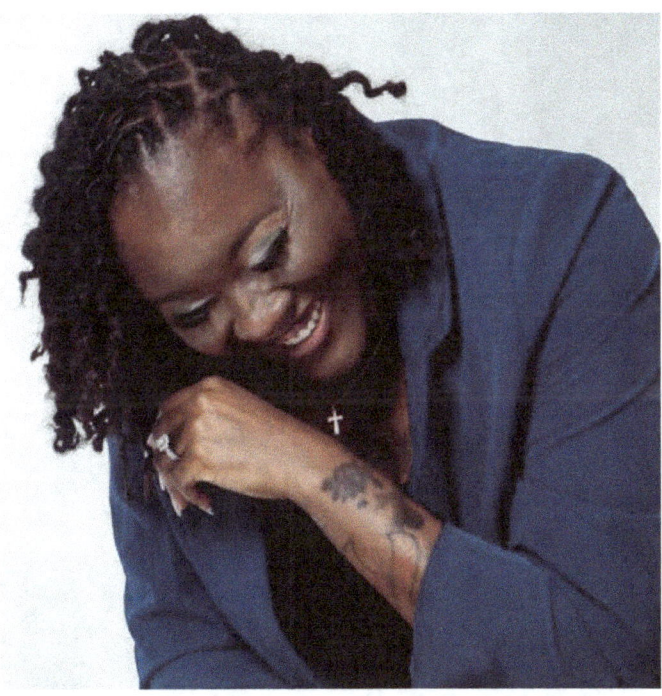

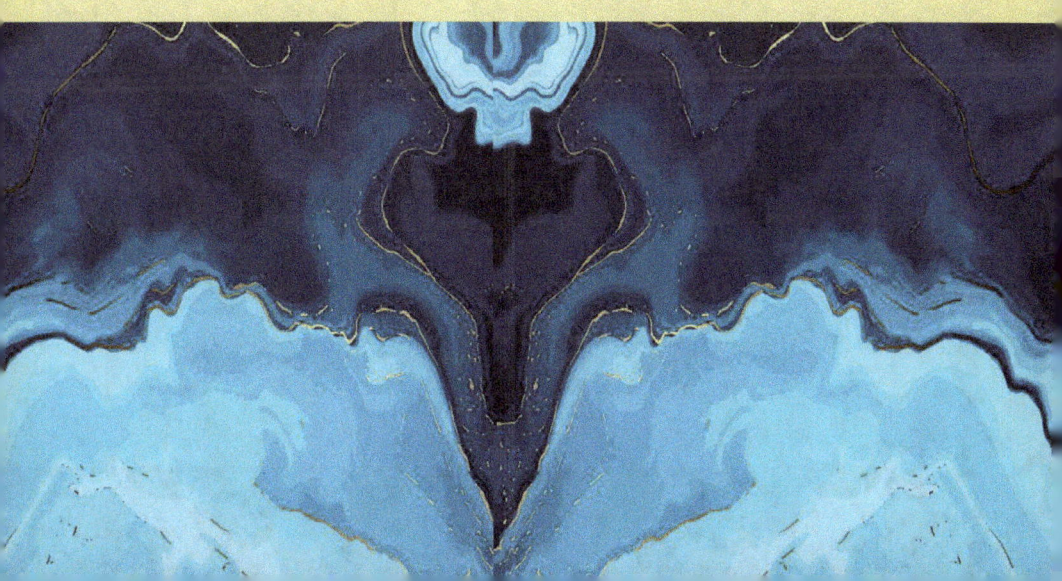

FOREWORD

la·bel (lā-bəl):
"*a classifying phrase or name applied to a person or thing, especially one that is inaccurate or restrictive.*"

The truth of the matter is: if the label we choose to wear is connected to a high-end designer or a luxury name-brand, then we flaunt it as if it defines our identities. However, if the label is synonymous with toxicity, trauma, or accountability – then we flee from it because we don't want to be identified or associated with such energy.

The saying "the first step to getting help is admitting you have a problem" is one of the realist statements because it speaks to *accountability!*

One of the problems we face when getting professional help is we typically look to place blame. We don't want to look at ourselves and find the fault in our actions or decisions that caused us to experience the trauma. The majority of time I hear people blaming the devil. Lord knows we give the devil way too much credit for situations that we create or can prevent. Think about it. The relationships that we stayed in knowing they were over but we continuously made excuses to stay.

Perhaps we're hopeful about the potential we see, or maybe just so comfortable with the convenient companionship that we find ourselves enduring pain longer than we needed to. Think about the times in which we were doing something that we know we had no business doing. We did it anyway – in the hopes of not getting caught or praying that the consequences would not circle around and haunt us. We as a people eat unhealthy, act unhealthy, and think unhealthy… yet wonder why we have health issues and troubled lifestyles.

No, I'm not saying that everything that happens in our lives is our fault – because we know that some things are out of our control. But what I am saying is that in order to take accountability for the things that happened in our lives we must:

1. Learn to love ourselves more than anything in this world.

2. Take a moment to self-reflect on the things that we can change, so moving forward doesn't come along with inflicting self-pain.

3. Accept the trauma that's happened in our lives and learn tools to heal from it – so that we're not carrying that pain into every other aspect of our lives.

Let's start with Step 1: learn to love yourself more than anything in this world. Now think about it – have you ever had a glass of water and someone asked for some? Because you had water in your glass, you were able to pour into theirs. Easy, right?

Now imagine having an empty glass and someone asking for water. How can you pour something that you don't have? This is key!

Check your relationships! Not just the intimate ones – but also the business-related, friendships and family dynamics. Some are not soul connections, some are not genuine, and some may be one-sided. These draining relationships leave you depleted and empty, with little to give anyone – especially *yourself*. These types of "*situationships*" or attachments are typical trauma-bonded relationships that you created to fill a void. They're caused by loneliness, lust, low self-esteem, and fear – all of which typically stem from trauma 99% of the time. Not all ties in your life actually *belong* in your life. You must quit binding yourself to these draining and unhealthy relationships. Some of these relationships are illusions of love used to replace the self-love that you deserve. When you learn to love yourself, then what you accept, allow to be poured into you, and even the outside love you desire will change for the better. Learn to love yourself more than anything in this world!

Now, let's circle to the second Step…

Take a moment to self-reflect on the things that we can change, so moving forward doesn't come along with inflicting self-pain. Imagine having a group of friends that shoplifts. You know they shoplift, yet you still decide to go with them to the mall. During this visit to the mall – they get caught and you become an accomplice. Do you think you shouldn't experience consequences?

I hope you were honest with yourself and said yes. (That's true accountability!)

Knowingly putting yourself in a situation you can be punished is nobody's fault but your own. This is an example when accountability and self-reflection are essential keys to growing. If you know that you're going into a place that's not safe, hanging with people that do bad things, are in "situationships" that are not beneficial, or know the things you are consuming are unhealthy for your body - when you still move forward in life doing these things that you know pose a risk, then it is only your fault that you allow yourself to be exposed to such consequences. Take a moment to self-reflect on the things we can change, so moving forward we aren't inflicting pain on ourselves.

And finally, Step 3.

We must accept the trauma that's happened in our lives and learn tools to heal from it, so that we're not carrying that pain into every other aspect of our lives. Unlike step two, there will be times in our lives where something will happen that is beyond our control. There may have been a person that has caused you harm, a diagnosis that affected your health, or you may have experienced the loss of a loved one that shifted your whole life. Those are all things that you cannot control. The best thing for us to do with those types of situations are to sit in them, deal with them and heal from them. We have no control over how a person treats us, but we have all the control over how we respond. In this day and age, no matter how healthy you eat, there is still a small chance that you may develop a disease, infection, or illness that may alter your livelihood.

Again, you have no control over that. One thing that is promised to us in this life is death, and no matter how painful it is – everyone is going to die. It happens to our loved ones when we least expect it at times. But even if we know that it's coming, it still hurts the same and we have no control over it. Again, what we *do* have is control over how we, ourselves, deal with those traumas. No one is to blame; there is no need to find fault. But the goal is to find a place of peace in knowing the incident is beyond our control. It's very inmportant to learn skills and acquire tools to process through the pain – so that we are not sitting around moping and feeling helpless or defeated about something we cannot change in the first place. This is **peace** in healing! There's a **weight lifted** when you can allow yourself to let go of the control you do not have. There is **joy** in knowing that through it all – you survived! If we can accept the trauma that's happened and learn tools to heal from it, we will find ourselves not carrying that pain into other aspects of our lives.

Life is not easy, so don't assume healing will be either. One thing's for sure though, the combination of **living life and healing** is priceless!

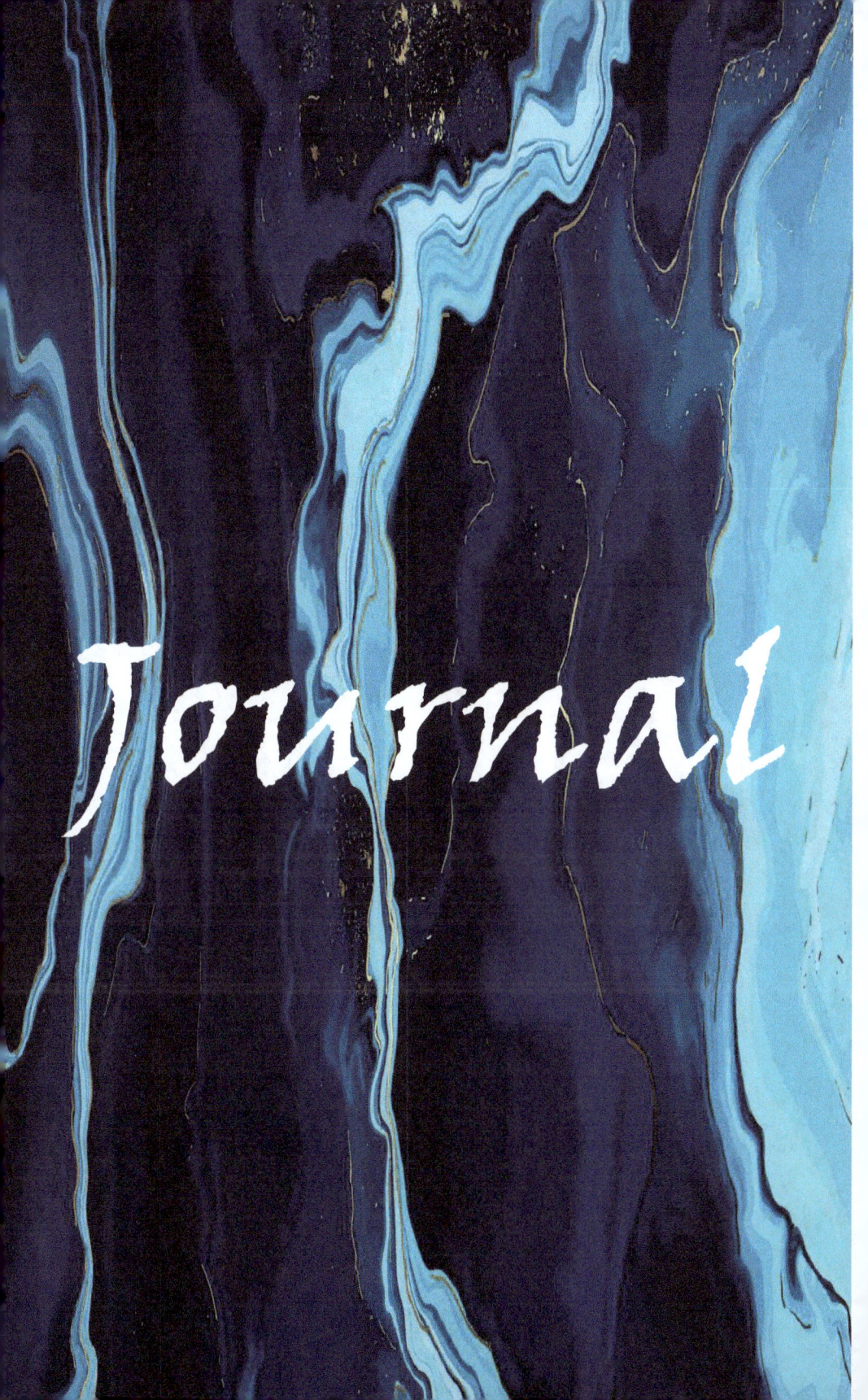

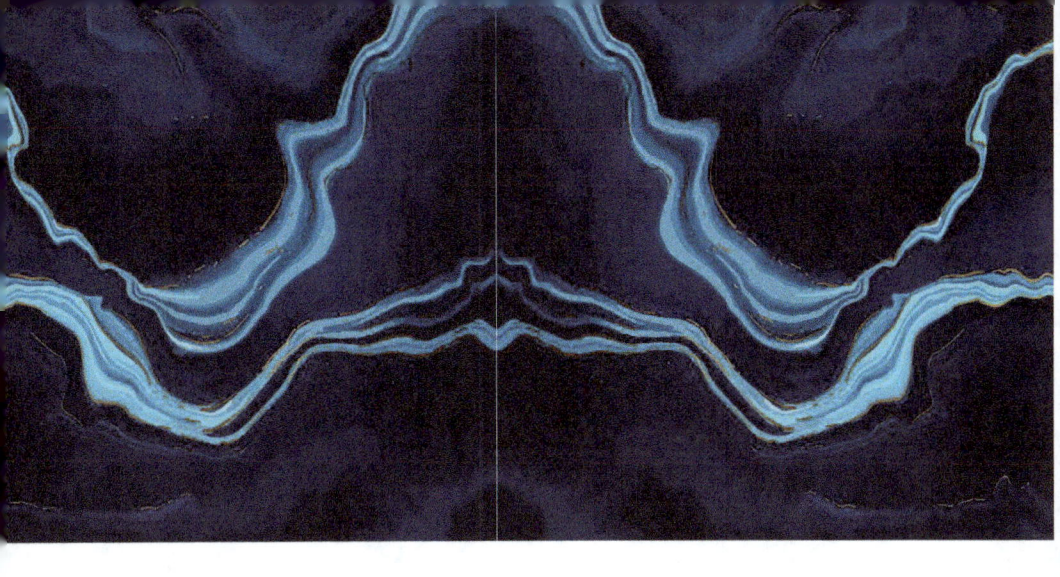

MY THOUGHTS

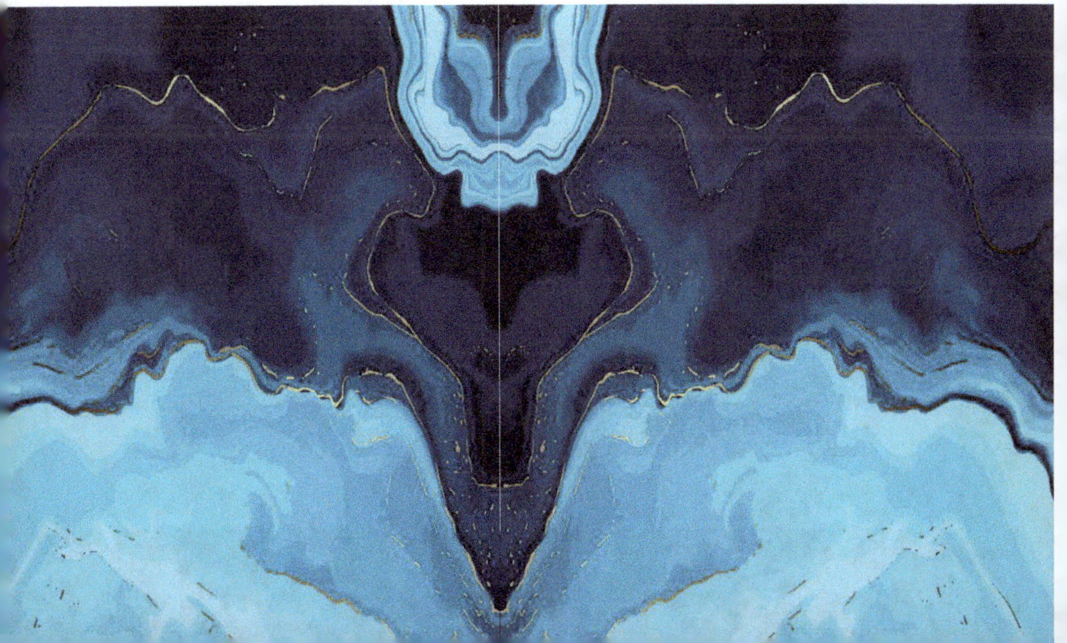

Day 0

My reason for writing this was simple: ***to inspire!***

I once had someone ask me why they should read MY STORY! My answer is, 'because I don't believe God had me go through all the things I went through to NOT help someone else.

Yes, my story may quite possibly be similar to many others', but the difference is my ability to articulate that pain in a way that resonates in their hearts while I convey strength through words. My journey is NOT my own. And I know that now because I used to question God, asking Him, "If You're so Holy, why would You allow your child to endure unnecessary pain? Why would You allow these things to happen to me if You knew it would have such an affect?"

And as I got older, I heard Him respond "Because had you not been through it and got through it, why would others trust me to help them through it without you praising me for being with you through it ALL!"

I remember a time when I was ANGRY with God and felt like I was a punishment child! Like I was suffering because of someone else's doings, but having been born, raised, and residing in Kansas City my whole life…I always had thoughts of relocating but the fear of starting over kept that from happening. UNTIL…

Just a few weeks into my second marriage, I was hit with devastating news from my (at the time) 8-year-old daughter that she had been molested! Having flashbacks from my own childhood trauma, I knew I had to ACT! I had to show my daughter that what happened to her

5

was not right and that the man who did it needed to be punished – by law, that is. Lord knows I wanted to take matters into my own hands, but I didn't. As a Black mother in a world that teaches us cops are bad, I wanted to give the justice system an opportunity to disprove that teaching for my daughter. So I called the police and filed a report.

My house was swarming with police officers, child protective services, and detectives for the rest of that week. Part of me seen why most people don't call the police and instead handle situations on their own – because the process was overwhelming. Having to witness my daughter relive the moment over and over as she repeatedly told the same story to multiple agencies…was the worst feeling I experienced as a mother. I felt hopeless but watching my daughter be so brave was inspiring. Her strength, her knowledge of right vs wrong, and her complete understanding of what was happening was astonishing to me! I was so proud of her. But truth is – the more the days passed, I became obsessed with finding this monster and handling him MYSELF! There were few words my husband could say that would comfort me. I was ANGRY! With the investigation going on and me trying to pretend things were normal, I ended up getting a call where I was offered a job in Florida. Nothing too amazing – but there was a pay increase from what I was currently making. I would be doing the same job as my then current position, but nonetheless it was an opportunity for a fresh start in a beautiful state away from this chaos!

I jumped on it. My husband – who had never traveled out of town the entirety of his adults years – was leery in the beginning. But I was eventually able to persuade him to risk the change with me. Two months later, we were moving to Florida…ready to start our new life as a married couple while giving my children an experience outside of Kansas City and for my daughter – a new start away from the trauma!

I never knew running from her trauma would create trauma for ME!

As I process through that trauma within this journal, I ask for your prayers that I continue my healing journey – because the road never ends!

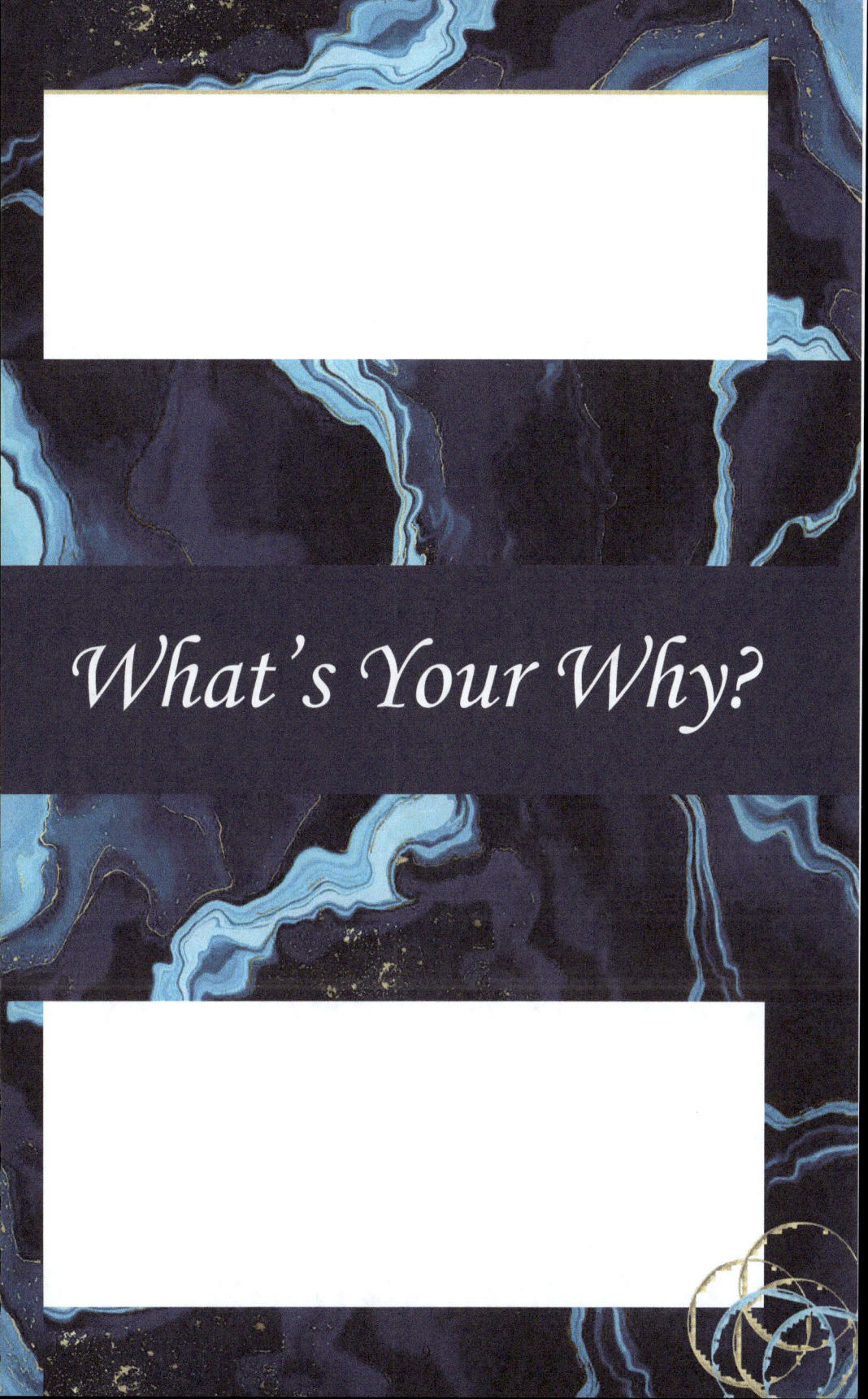

What's Your Why?

Personal Journaling

MY REASON FOR STARTING THIS JOURNAL

_____

_____

_____

_____

_____

_____

MY BIGGEST FEAR OR HESITATION IN THIS JOURNEY

_____

_____

_____

_____

_____

_____

WHAT I HOPE TO ACCOMPLISH IN SPITE MY FEAR

_____

_____

_____

_____

PEOPLE I WILL CALL IF I GET OVERWHELMED

_____

_____

_____

_____

_____

_____

PEOPLE I WILL CALL IF I NEED ENCOURAGEMENT

_____

_____

_____

_____

_____

_____

PLACES I WILL GO FOR RELEASE OR TO ESCAPE
CAN BE SONGS, MOVIES, PLACES, OR ACTIVITIES/HOBBIES

_____

_____

_____

_____

ADVICE TO MYSELF / AFFIRMATIONS / SELF-ENCOURAGEMENT

TAKE A PICTURE OF YOURSELF AND PLACE IT HERE.
OR TAKE A SELFIE AND SAVE IT IN YOUR FAVORITES.
WRITE THE DATE BELOW SO YOU CAN FIND THE SELFIE
LATER FOR REFERENCE.

DATE & SIGN:

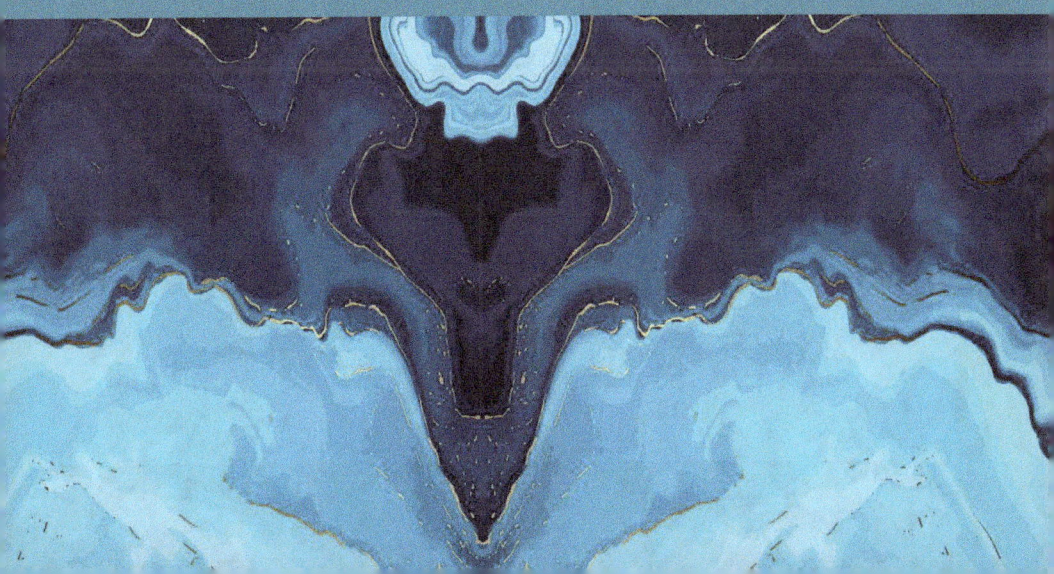

SELF CARE

What is Self-Care?

As mentioned in the foreword, self-love is critical. The person that you committed to doing this journal with is YOU. And there is no way that you can begin to SIT IN YO SHIT if you don't show kindness to yourself. This starts in the form of self-care.

Self-care is the act of creating, prioritizing, and providing intimate space with your thoughts, feelings, emotions, prayers, and honestly, your _essence_. It can be so easy to prioritize work, relationships, household chores, volunteering, children, and family that we often leave out ourselves. I mean – it's easier to do so because we can _see_ them.

Think about it – very infrequently do you interact or prioritize the things that you cannot physically see. And since we don't walk around with mirrors hovering in front of us to constantly see OURSELVES – it can be easy to forget.

For some of us, looking in the mirror can be a reminder of all things we have been trying to run from, including past traumas…

But it doesn't have to be. Imagine finding a huge. diamond in the mud or better yet, in a pile of _shit_. You see the glimmers – but in order to grab the diamond, you have to stick your hand literally in some shit to pull it out. But with a little pull and tug, some cleaning, maybe even sanitizing along with a polishing treatment…you will have unveiled a treasure.

That is what we call _tender, loving care_. We owe it to ourselves and our loved ones to create a space of self-TLC. Trust me, this is no easy task. In fact, I struggle with it daily and many times I fail. And that's okay because I bounce back and remember the commitment that I owe to myself. You just committed to you, too. (If you thought I'd let you skip past p. 14, think again! Take the time now to go back and sign. Remember, we are all about ACCOUNTABILITY here.)

Throughout this journal are various self-care exercises to help you along the road towards self-TLC. I encourage you to do them in a safe space or place that you can make your own. If you don't have a room, get creative! Use your car, bathroom, a park, your bed – WHEREVER! Just find…a…place.

To accompany each exercise, take 20-30 minutes for yourself, if you can. That time can be immediately before or after you complete each exercise. If 20-30 minutes is difficult to carve out, then take 5 minutes for yourself to just pray or do an activity that you love.

The point is *to start living out the commitment to yourself.*

YOU are the CEO of your life and you owe it to yourself to show up to for your shift at Me, Myself, and I, LLC.

5 Minute Gratitude Exercise

___/___/___

S M T W TH F S

Breathe before writing

INHALE
EXHALE
INHALE
EXHALE
INHALE
EXHALE

3 best things about today

Things you're grateful for today

* _____
* _____
* _____
* _____
* _____

Today's Highlight

Describe today in a drawing

Things that you learned

_____
_____
_____
_____

Today's Affirmation:

_____

CHILDHOOD TRAUMA

Day 1
What happened???

Have you ever just woke up on a random day, looked around your room, and asked yourself, "What the fuck happened?" Everything before the day you woke up seems like a blur. Could it be memory loss? Maybe it's just *wanting* to lose the memory of the reality. Most of the time it is hard to begin the healing process because we want to ignore or bury the trauma.

The only thing I could remember was one day I was happy, then the next day we were arguing all the time about nothing. Literally, nothing. One day it was about dead fish, the next it was about me going to work in all black. Majority of the arguments made no sense. They eventually started to drain me and had me questioning my marriage as a whole. I didn't realize the signs even then; it just all seemed like frustration trying to adjust to the move.

I made excuses for him. "Maybe he misses his kids and family." "Maybe it's because he's having a hard time finding the right job." Never did I think it would have been what it became!

Take this moment of sitting in your shit and ask yourself what REALLY happened. What is it that really has me feeling this way? Identify the situation and identify each emotion you're feeling as you think about this situation.

Day 2

How the FAWK did I get here?

Trauma rewrites our DNA. Forget who our parents are, when trauma strikes we become a new person. And that person is alive until we take an active stance on healing and put that trauma to rest. We must heal and evolve above the pain that holds us down knowingly and unknowingly.

We often use quotes such as, "it's just who I am" as though it's a justifiable statement to get a pass on our behaviors/thoughts. The inner child in us wants to heal. The pain causes temper tantrums that spill out into our actions and behaviors. When we can have effective, healthy communications about our emotions , manage our anger, not have to seek sexual pleasures to feel good about ourselves, or not resort to alcohol/drugs to numb the pain, we're moving in the right direction. When we don't have to engage in risky behaviors just to experience an internal adrenaline rush that gives us a high that pleases our soul – that's when we are actively making a conscience decision to heal. As much as we hate to admit it, most of who we are today is based on our childhood.

As I reflect on the cycles of my relationship choices, they all fall back on voids I'm trying to fill from childhood. Wanting to be protected, wanting to feel validated and be reassured that I'm ENOUGH and worth fighting for! All that unhealed trauma caused me to ignore vital signs that lead to toxic relationships.

27

Today we won't focus on the NOW, but more so on the THEN. The "THEN" will help us identify why things are happening in the "NOW".

Use this time to write about what you remember growing up. The good, bad, and ugly!

Day 3

Triggering Trauma

Alllllllllll my life I've been broke, naw naw for real!! I wasn't going to include this in the book but hell y'all getting the real me and as I was typing this – this is what I thought! That song popped in my head when I typed the word "Alllllll". But seriously.....

"Alllll my life I had to fight."

Lol, no seriously. Movie trivia? If you said *Color Purple*, then you're right! I felt that line and could relate! Can you?

I literally had to fight for attention, fight to be loved, fight to prove my love, fight for acceptance! No wonder I stayed in an abusive relationship for 10 years, right?

Well, when I got in my second marriage, he showed me a different fight! He fought for ME! Not physically but when we broke up he was adamant to get me back. So adamant that he popped up at my house, called all the time, and even randomly rode past my parents' house. At first it was irritating. I even told my daddy to ask him to stop but it became "cute". Not really but definitely attractive to my trauma in a toxic way that created a trigger inside of me. The behavior sparked a feeling that made me feel valuable, needed, and worthy.

Oooo I thought that was love and FINALLY – I found someone that believed I was worthy enough to fight for instead of fighting me!

Not knowing my trauma blinded me to a red flag and symptom of his diagnosis.

As a child, I never felt accepted by other kids and when bad things happened to me…I never had anyone willing to fight or go to bat for me. I never had anyone go to war behind me. Rarely did I feel protected and I always felt like I was out in this world alone.

It wasn't until much later that I realized my lack of feeling protected as a child consequently blinded me from my present day reality. *Him* fighting for me wasn't a *healthy* fight, but instead was a red flag of a mental illness symptom. He was very insecure; always thought people were out to get him. And when I broke up with him, even though he possibly loved me, his desire to control the situation and have his way was the motivating reason he would fight to get me back.

During the breakup, I rekindled a flame with an old friend. That provoked my ex to new levels in his mission to get me back, as he then became obsessed with my new boyfriend and even started calling me to talk about him. Again, my trauma found that as a cute form of jealously! He would call and give me identifying characteristics or other details of my new boyfriend, clueing me in that he discovered who it was.

"Awww, you found out who I'm dating?" was my thought when he would call. My ex was adamant to get me back! He even had his sister call and advocate for him. He made up lies about leaving things at my house to see if I would allow him to come over. I declined every time but he was persistent. It sometimes created discomfort in my new relationship but due to other reasons, that relationship didn't last long. And my ex was still hanging around, fighting for my attention. Then he left a voicemail crying and *that's* what got me! I'm such a sucker for men being emotional. So I finally gave in and called him back. Months later we were married. All these things were red flags and I missed them because I wanted to be *fought for* so bad.

It's easy to blame others, but we have to recognize when we create our own storms by ignoring the warning signs of bad weather!

Take this time to identify the red flags that you may have possibly missed that led to your current trauma. Once you identify those red flags, reflect on your childhood or previous traumas to see how ignoring them brought you false comfort.

Finally, write about a time where you mistakenly accepted a red flag because you were blinded by trauma.

Day 4

This shit is hard, huh?

Man, by the time I got here, I was emotionally drained! I found more people to point the finger at, more people to be mad at. I was angry with the whole world! Looking back on my childhood trauma, I was mad at the people that was supposed to protect me as a CHILD! I was a freaking kid and had no business prices being involved in adult bullshit! Shame on them! Shame on the people that took advantage of me! Shame on the people that couldn't look beyond my acting out and see that I was a child hurting on the inside! Nobody SAW ME! Nobody realized I was hurting, so from that point forward I was MY KEEPER! My protector, my EVERYTHING!

That was a helluva load to carry!

As you begin to heal, it is important that you remove some of the load. Take off some of those capes you wear being your own superhero!

Self-care is an essential part of healing. You have to be intentional about being KIND to yourself! LOVING YOURSELF! And giving yourself GRACE! We do not know everything – and that's okay!

For all the love I gave out to people in hopes of getting it back, I consciously made a decision to start giving that same love and energy to *me* FIRST!

Today, take time for yourself.

Breathe!! No – like seriously – BREATHE right now!

Follow these directions but *read* them first! Be sure to perform each step!!

- *Go into a room where you can be alone*
  - *Turn the lights off*
  - *Remove your socks/shoes*
- *Rub your feet on the ground. Get in tune with the room, the darkness, and the silence*
- *Take 5 deep breaths – inhale in for 5 seconds, then exhale for 5 seconds*
  - *Sit in the complete silence for 60 seconds*

Do this now before coming back to the next page to journal. Don't cheat!! Aht Aht!! Do not flip the page until you've completed this exercise!!!

*Welcome back. Now you can turn the page.

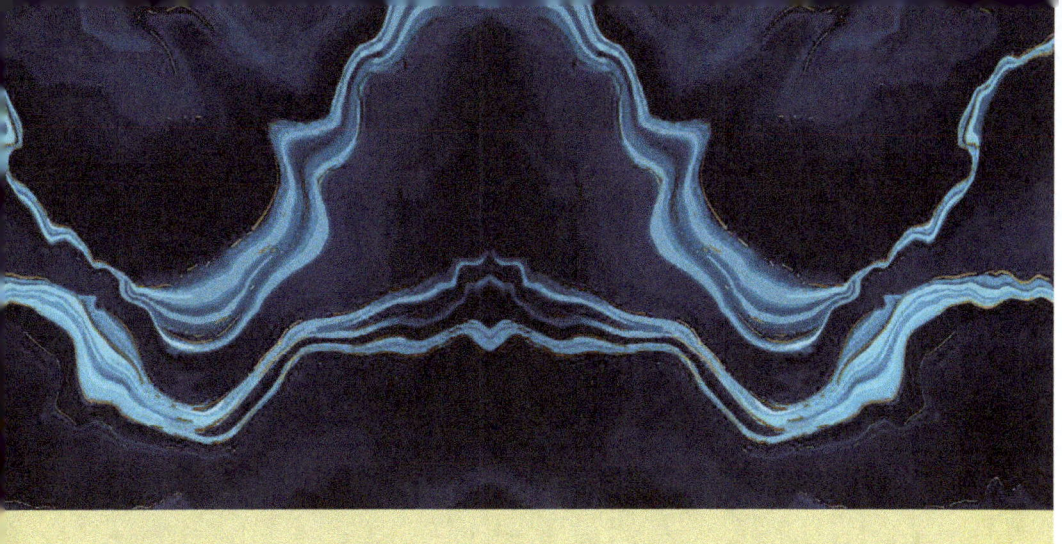

SELF CARE

Journal about what you felt sitting in the darkness, in complete silence. Did you hear things from other rooms? How did you *feel?* Did your body respond in a way you can explain?

Sometimes, taking the time to sit still and be intentional in doing *nothing* allow us to hear the things around us more clearly. For the next week, I encourage you to do this breathing exercise before bed! It really helped with my insomnia and nightmares. Praying it'll do some good for you as well!

Tonight – take a warm bubble bath, drink a glass of wine, and relax your mind! You deserve it!

Feelings Grid

Intensity of Feelings	HAPPY	SAD	ANGRY	CONFUSED
High	Elated Excited Overjoyed Thrilled Exuberant Ecstatic Fired Up Delighted	Depressed Heartbroken Alone Hurt Unwanted Dejected Hopeless Sorrowful Crushed	Furious Enraged Outraged Aggravated Irate Seething	Bewildered Trapped Troubled Desperate Lost
Medium	Cheerful Up Good Relieved Satisfied Pleased	Disappointed Down Upset Distressed Regret Left Out	Upset Mad Annoyed Frustrated Agitated Hot Disgusted	Disorganized Foggy Misplaced Disoriented Mixed Up Lost
Low	Glad Satisfied Pleasant Fine Mellow	Unhappy Moody Blue Sorry Bad Dissatisfied	Perturbed Uptight Dismayed Irritated Discontent	Unsure Puzzled Bothered Uncomfortable Undecided Baffled Perplexed

Day 5

Nobody cares as much as you...

Have you ever sat on the front row at a homegoing and listened to people say over and over, "if you need anything, I'm here?" I despise funerals for that reason. In the moment, everybody is readily available. They have all the stories and support. They're ready to bring all the meals. But when that casket closes, everybody goes on about their own lives. Some may check-in from time to time – mainly on holidays or special occasions/anniversaries. But because it wasn't them...some people simply *forget!*

The same goes for trauma – when it's fresh, everyone is around. They're making promises to be there, saying how they're only a phone call away, etc. The truth is: as the days pass, most loved ones carry on about their life. All the while, you're still dealing with the pain, memories, trauma, grief, and loss...left to readjust to your life's new reality.

I remember wishing someone would call and check on me, ask me if I'm okay. No one ever did. If *I* took the initiative to reach out, friends and family would then offer a listening ear – reassuring encouragement or maybe even a thoughtful social media post from time to time. But it was nothing compared to hoping someone *else* took the initiative to do the wellness check. The harsh reality is...life DOES go on. It's okay to **sit in yo shit** when the emotions, thoughts, and pains become overwhelming! But DON'T *STAY* THERE!

At times, I would wake up in full-blown sweats from nightmares! I started working from home because driving down the street and seeing a white Jeep would send me into a full blown panic attack! Anytime a court date was approaching, my sleep would be off that entire week prior – leaving me restless and irritable. But no one noticed. When you're typically the STRONG one, it especially goes unnoticed! I hated that people went on with life, thinking mine was back to normal. I hated that it wasn't! I had many moments where I battled my thoughts – being sad about the situation one day, having pity on him the next, and then being angry with him on other days! Trauma really sends you on an emotional rollercoaster!

It is important that we identify our emotions during this process.

Use this time to journal about what you feel in THIS moment!

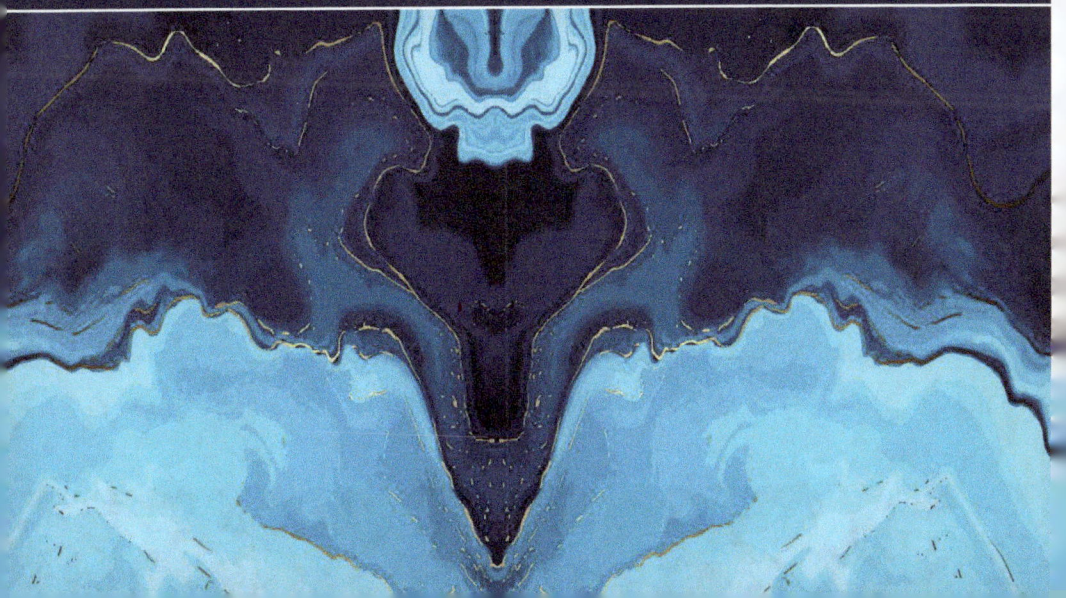

THE SITUATION

Day 6

The Day

After nine months of marriage and a five month process of relocating to our new home in a new state, I thought my life was really beginning. I had a great job, nice home, and a beautiful car. My kids were happy and I thought my husband and I were, too. The week leading up to **The Day**, I had to travel back to my hometown to bury my dad's only sister. Losing her was hard because she was like a bonus mother to me. She helped raise me and all my memories about her were from when I was a tiny tot. She helped teach me how to cook. She had a cleaning company and taught me how to clean. Hell, she was the closest woman to me on my dad's side.

I thought my spouse would be sympathetic to my loss; he was the complete opposite. During the time I was away for the funeral, my husband created narratives in his mind that got the best of him. He constantly called to listen in on my background. To appease him, I allowed it. He then sent very distasteful texts as I slept the evening before I came back home, assuming I was with a man.

The morning I returned home from my aunt's funeral – my husband, protector, and friend was so convinced that I had been cheating on him…that he pulled out a gun and threatened to take my life. This was **the day** my whole life shattered into a million pieces…

"Here I am again, having to face yet *another* divorce, another FAILED marriage. What the fawk is wrong with me?!"

Use this time to vividly write out your situation/trauma. Be descriptive! Include details using all of your five senses (see, hear, taste, smell & feel).

Get it out your system!

Day 7

You are not at fault...

Oh – now that you've sat, identified what happened, and realized how you got there – it's a hard pill to swallow saying you're at fault, right???

Now understand me clearly – you're never at fault for any abuse, harm or pain done to you!

When I say you're 'at fault', I'm saying take accountability in the fact that you ignored certain signs or symptoms that may have lead you to this place. No, I would never condone the things that my ex did to me or make excuses for that to happen to anyone else. I don't care if you got a smart mouth. I don't care if you spend bill money. I don't care if they were on drugs or if somebody was cheating. Regardless of the situation, nobody has the right to hurt another human being. So, if that happened to you – from the bottom of my heart, I apologize and pray for your healing. I pray healing for who hurt you and I pray that you find forgiveness in your heart so that you can move on. But no matter what happened to you or the trauma it caused…it is your responsibility to heal! Even if you didn't get an apology, that doesn't mean you don't have an opportunity to forgive and move on in your healing journey.

Use this time to identify any trauma from your childhood that may have impacted your decision-making leading up to this situation.

Examples:
Choosing the wrong people out of need for acceptance
Not setting healthy boundaries from fear of not being accepted/respected

Day 8

What is love?

What is love? Baby don't hurt me, don't hurt me…no more… - Haddawa

Write down another song about love that comes to your mind.

_____

Now, let's define love. In the space below, write what love is to you.

_____

The infamous scripture often quoted at weddings and used to describe love is *1st Corinthians 13:4-5,* which says:

4 Love is patient, love is kind. It does not envy, it does not boast, it is not proud. **5** It does not dishonor others, it is not self-seeking, it is not easily angered, it keeps no record of wrongs.

I quoted this scripture in my vows. And I meant them. This scripture was the representation of the man I was marrying. He was patient with me. Even when I was a firecracker, he was always kind to me. Never cursed me out, called me out my name, or put his hands on me. He was definitely a breath of fresh air from my last husband! Even when I was upset, it took a lot for me to anger him and when I did – he still showed self-control and calmness. I mean, to be honest, I think there was only one time I really triggered him.

He meant everything to me. I was anxious to start a life with this tall, handsome, calm-spirited, well-cooking man. He seemed to be everything my busy self needed. He calmed me down and I introduced him to a different world. I thought it was a match made in Heaven, so no wonder I didn't blink twice on my wedding day. HE was who I wanted and I had him.

Never in a million years did I expect the "representation of (that) man" to go away. But, boy oh boy, the representation hid him well. So well that even my family who knew his past trusted that this newer version of him just might be proof that he was a different person now. Both *my family* and *his* believed this so much that they decided not to warn me of the "old him".

I trusted him. I was happy to be his wife. I was ready to share my life with him. I loved him…

But now I find myself singing…

"What's love got to do, got to do with it? What's love but a secondhand emotion?" (in my Tina Turner voice)

Love don't keep a marriage! Trust, honesty, commitment, communication and TOGETHERNESS does. And it has to be coming from BOTH parties 100%.

Here I am, being called his "QUEEN" – with him feeling like he couldn't live life without me. All to the point where he could have taken my life along with his! Thank God that chapter wasn't destined that morning.

How do you love someone you can't trust, when you say you love them enough to commit a lifetime to them?

Some other definitions of love are:

- A willingness to prioritize another's well-being or happiness above your own.
- Extreme feelings of attachment, affection, and need.
- Dramatic, sudden feelings of attraction and respect.
- A fleeting emotion of care, affection, and like.

The first one stands out to me because it implies a selfless act and not an emotion – making 'love' a verb, instead of a noun.

In order for love to be beneficial to a MARRIAGE, it has to be an action. An unconditional, selfless action that focuses on another as opposed to self.

Anytime love is used in a marriage as an emotion it becomes and shall remain *conditional*. When it's based on how the other person makes YOU FEEL…it essentially makes the love 'wavering'.

I was thinking I knew love, was love, and *gave* love – but I was blinded by what I *wanted* more than what was *present*.

Do I believe he didn't love me? No, but his illness hindered him from being able to love in the healthiest, purest form of how God described love to be.

Describe the confusion in processing what you thought was love when it turned into pain.

Day 9

Fuck the 5 Steps of Grief

THEY SAY….

The five steps of grief are:
1. Denial and Isolation
2. Anger
3. Bargaining
4. Depression
5. Acceptance

Who made this list and gave it an order?

My steps of grief have been:

Denial and isolation, anger, confusion, depression, bargaining, anger, denial, more anger, more depression. Hell, I'm yet to experience *acceptance*.

For the first time dealing with ANY trauma – I've actually **sat in this shit**, felt this pain, fought my thoughts, beat myself up, and asked myself so many questions. I blamed others; I blamed myself.

Blaming myself was the hardest place to come out of. Every time I thought of the situation, it always fell back on me.

How could he try to kill me? "You should have proved you wasn't cheating on him, Devin!"

Why didn't he love me enough to protect me from him? "You chose him, Devin!"

He could have told me about his mental illness. "Did you give him a safe space to feel comfortable telling you this, Devin?"

No matter what he did, I made it my fault. I put myself in harm's way. I put my parents in harm's way. I could have put my children in harm's way and I ruined his life!!

But did I really?

I can't plan and be in control of ALL things, right? Hell, I still don't know. But what I do know is that I'm alive, my parents are alive, my children are alive, and we are all safe!! There's a blessing in that and that alone!!!

In order to pull myself out the darkness, I had to counteract every negative thought with a positive affirmation.

I had to look myself in the mirror and tell myself,

"Now look here...that's enough of the pity party. Time to level up and focus on getting out of this shit! It's ok to have bad days, but ain't no more bad *weeks*."

Write down how you remember or are currently processing your steps of grief. It's totally okay if you repeat a few steps but write down what you remember.

Day 10

Sit Cho ASS Down!

I would have never known relocating would turn out to be such a blessing for me. I originally thought this was a new beginning for my marriage and children – but this definitely helped ME!

I often asked myself if my ex-husband's true self would have shown had we stayed in our hometown. I was told that his "episodes" appeared because he was out of his comfort zone. I was also told that at some point his true colors would have exposed themselves and without medication and/or therapy, it was only a matter of time before I experienced his illness firsthand.

I know for a fact that had we still lived in our hometown after this trauma happened, I would have surrounded myself with friends. I would have made an excuse to hang out partying…just so I didn't have to feel this, deal with this, and heal from this.

There is a benefit to being surrounded by love – but there is also a greater benefit being able to sit alone in your shit and REALLY deal with trauma!

The days leading up to this trauma were already overwhelming, to say the least. I've never been the one to handle death well. Even though my aunt had shown signs that the end was near…it still hurt. While at the memorial service I remember FaceTiming him to reassure him of my whereabouts after he stated that "my aunt hadn't passed and I was really in town to see my ex". Strangely, I didn't even acknowledge the statement. I just made sure to prove the truth and that still didn't work.

During the entire 4-day trip, I found myself battling with him over HIS insecurities! That, in turn, made the grieving process for my aunt that much harder.

Majority of the time when I'm faced with having to grieve, I intentionally make myself busy so I don't have to feel the sensation. Ironically, dealing with his insecurities was a great distraction from mourning, but grief still resurfaced later.

What things do you notice yourself doing to avoid feeling or dealing with pain, trauma, or any stressors?

THE MAN IN THE MIRROR

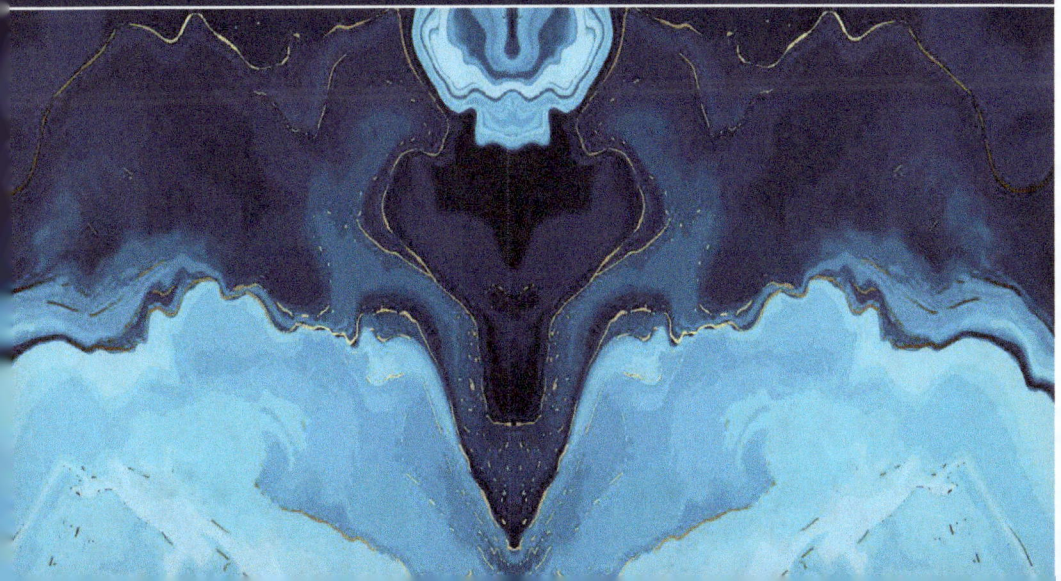

Day 11

Fuck Feelings

After all the processing, playing the blame game, crying, and being angry – I'm finally at a point where I'm TIRED! I'm so tired of being tired. Feeling hurt and confused; mad and sad. Worthless and disrespected. Not good enough and too good at the same time. Dumb, stupid, naive, and used…

Have you ever faked having confidence? I mean, walked in a room – head held high and nose to the sky? Embracing every foot of height, every curve, and loving all your Blackness – but deep inside feeling lanky, too black, and sometimes ugly??

I've lived a life so fake, I don't know what's real. Do I love myself? What is love? How can you ask for the unknown?

I'm a piece of work!!

I wanna know what love isssss! I want you to shoowww me...

Song trivia?? Lol if you said *Foreigner* then you're right! I know I had to Google it, too, but those lyrics hit!

Google the lyrics to this song; listen to it!

Based on how you've received love, how would you define it? Write down the ideal type of the love you want to experience.

Day 12

The pain is for a moment…

I heard a quote that says, "the pain is for a moment, but the healing lasts a lifetime."

We really have to be *intentional* about allowing ourselves to heal and process through pain. So often we get complacent in hurting because it becomes the new norm, but it's not healthy. With healing comes PEACE, and it's critical that we protect our peace at all costs!

And sometimes you have to be selfish to protect your peace.

Use this day to do something for you! Take yourself out to lunch, go to the movies, go get a manicure/pedicure, or take a walk in the park...

JUST DO SOMETHING FOR *YOU*.

And then come back and tell us about it.

Day 13

Closure

I read a post on social media that said, "the disrespect was all the closure you needed."

BULLSHIT.

I NEED TO KNOW WHY, HOW, WHAT – EVERYTHING!

The morning I returned home from my aunt's homegoing service, my ex-husband was still under the impression that I had went back to Kansas City to cheat on him. When I woke up to get ready for work, he woke up ready for war! He jumped out of bed as soon as my alarm went off – yelling derogatory names, being extremely disrespectful, and expressing his thoughts on my "cheating". He expressed within that argument that our marriage was over and he couldn't trust me anymore!

Now, for those who don't know me, I can be pretty snappy with my words. But this particular morning, I remember feeling an energy that reassured me to *stay calm*. It was weird because with all the arguing that had taken place over the past few months, I hadn't necessarily been quick to keep my mouth closed. But this morning something told me to do so. I went to the shower and he came into the bathroom, snatched the curtains back and continued to argue with me. It almost felt like he was antagonizing or trying to provoke me. Even with our previous fights, I'd never seen him act THIS way. He was very verbally aggressive and that wasn't like him. Him noticing that I wasn't responding angered him more and he began making comments about my parents, whom I'm sure he knew I'd defend to the ends of earth. However, I didn't want to defend them in this moment. I wanted him to realize that they were *sleeping in our home.*

Unbeknownst to him, when we were flying home to FL the night before, my parents and I missed our flight causing us to get home at 1am. They were supposed to sign documents the next day in the city they were moving to, but plans changed when we had to catch a later flight. They didn't want me driving home alone, so instead of dropping them off – they just came home with me and spent the night. When my ex started yelling disrespectful things in reference to my parents, I instantly tried to inform him that they were sleeping in our home so that my parents didn't hear. At some point in the argument, he made a statement about my mother that stung and I responded about him not being raised by his mother. And that's when he raised the gun up to me with the beam on my heart and I heard him say "say one more thing and I'ma kill you". My heart stopped and everything became a blur…

Thankfully I was able to get out of that situation alive and the police took him into custody. We had our first court date and things still didn't feel real. A day or so later, I got a call from his sister and cousin. They proceeded to give me news about his diagnosis that I had no knowledge of prior to our marriage. THIS was my first time hearing that my husband at the time was diagnosed with Schizophrenia and they insisted that, as his wife, I should help him! I took that as the "drop-the-charges because he is sick and your life means nothing" plea. Why tell me now? What if this had turned out differently? With them knowing he suffered from this illness, how would they have felt?

I was so enraged by his actions and everybody's willingness to help keep his secret that I felt everybody that knew owed me an apology! I wanted apologies and the truth!!!

Did HE, not the *representation* of him, really love me? Was he sorry? And how could he do this to me, his WIFE?

What things did *you* need to find closure from your trauma/pain?

Day 14

Welcome Back

You checked out, huh?

By this time I had. I was tired of crying, tired of thinking, tired of FEELING.

ALL I wanted was to seem normal again.

I checked out by this time in my journey and if you didn't do the same in *this* moment, maybe you did earlier in the book. The only thing that's important is that now you are back – reading this page! I know it's hard, but you're almost there. Almost through the journal, but still on the journey! And that is commendable! Pat yourself on the back!

I told you this journey wouldn't be easy. Sometimes it takes days or months to get back on the track of healing, but don't delay the process too far out!

Give yourself grace to do ABSOLUTELY NOTHING. Don't think, don't feel, DON'T process – just *rest!*

Rest in knowing that regardless of it all – YOU ARE STILL HERE!!

Today is a free day.

Write down something or write down nothing. But *at least* jot something down to express gratitude because we are alive. 💚

Day 15

Reality Check

This was the hardest pill to swallow: admitting that I'M TOXIC!

I just realized it. And the crazy thing is, I'm quick to say that about *other* people.

The fact that I haven't healed causes me to respond to other situations based on MY trauma. There are times I'm very aggressive, stubborn, and sometimes completely narcissistic! I've had my share of playing the victim when I knew I was dead ass wrong. My actions were toxic enough to deserve to lose my life. However, I must admit I've definitely been wrong before – a lot of times.

It wasn't until I dealt with a person that was healthy in areas where I was unhealthy and they could call me out when I was wrong that I truly realized how toxic I could be.

It hurt like hell to face that truth. With all my counseling and all the people around me that held me accountable – it took an intimate, yet safe relationship for someone to point out my wrongs in a way where I was able to receive it.

If you ask that person, I'm sure they'd say I fought them a lot. Not physically, but I definitely pressed issues I should have left alone. I argued when I should have kept my mouth closed; I pushed good people away! I'm sure my actions were very draining to loved ones. Hell, my actions drained *me* plenty of times. I've hurt myself by causing pain to others that I love. They always say the first step in getting help is *admitting you have a problem!*

Today, be real with yourself! We've talked about how others have done us wrong and how we've been treated. But we can't forget *our* roles in this!

Write down your flaws, your areas that could use improvement, and how you may have added to the situation...

Day 16

Dealing is Healing

Looking within is almost always the hardest thing to do – because the "victim" in us wants to point blame. We want to find peace in identifying who or what hurt us, instead of knowing that true self-accountability is the very thing that keeps us from making the same mistakes.

Self-reflection helps us to process who we are or once were. We're then able to compare *that* person to who we *want* to be. It gives us a map with directions to the final destination of *healing*.

While healing, we tend to juggle a lot. We sometimes become submerged in the pain and guilt. The truth is – we CAN'T stay there. Sometimes when the weight gets heavy, our thoughts become blurred and our path gets dark…but remember to *stay the course!*

I always say it's better to be *proactive* versus *reactive*.

Use this time to write out a list of things that you can do when you are feeling down, people who will hold you accountable to being still, or social events that can encourage the healing process. (You'll need this throughout your healing journey for sure.)

Compare this list to your list from Day 0. Has your perspective on healing, the things you need, or the people you plan to call changed based on your journey to this point?

It's ok if it has! Consider it a good thing that you are identifying your needs for YOUR HEALING! And another thing, be okay with knowing the list may change due to growth. Everything isn't for everybody!

Examples:

- listen to music
- attend church
- dine in at your favorite restaurant

Day 17

Self-Reflection

Self-reflection is my favorite place. ♡

This is where I start realizing that people's actions have nothing to do with me and everything to do with their hurt and their problems.

It has *nothing* to do with *my worth!!*

I'm thankful for this time of healing, reflection, growth, and CREATING. ♡ ◇

Now that we've talked about forgiving others and ourselves, looked back over our childhood trauma, and thought about how those pains open doors to new pains in the future – what have we learned?

Write a letter to your version of self from a week *before* your trauma. Advise yourself on the situation that's going to happen. Encourage yourself to heal through the pain. And forecast what your future, healed self will be like.

Day 18

How dare you pull a Me on me?

Oftentimes we hold on so tight to the things we should've let go of long before the pain struck. We so badly desire to see potential and hope that we end up staying – all while praying for change. We be sitting up wishing upon a star night after night after night…knowing that we aren't seeing any changes, but we stay anyway. And honestly, because of those decisions – we are the ones to blame for the pain and trauma. We breathe, eat, piss, and digest so much shit that we are now *living in a funk* – figuratively and literally speaking! Have you ever asked yourself *why*? Have you ever thought it's because we don't value, love, and forgive ourselves? We continue to put ourselves in situations where we're comfortable and complacent in pain because that's the only thing we know. We allow people to treat us poorly because it's a representation of how we treat *ourselves*. The only reason we eventually walk away is because the pain becomes more than what we'd put on ourselves. Once we are done hurting, we say to ourselves, 'Aht aht – can't nobody hurt me worse than me!' Then, we finally find the motivation to pack up our shit and walk away!

Right now – I need you to get off your high horse and *sit the hell down*. It's time that you do something for yourself! Write yourself an apology letter – asking for forgiveness for whatever your heart needs to heal from. Ask yourself for forgiveness for putting yourself through things when you knew you deserved better. Ask yourself for forgiveness for allowing people to diminish the value in you that God created.

Letter of Apology

_____
_____
_____
_____
_____
_____
_____
_____
_____
_____
_____
_____
_____
_____
_____
_____
_____
_____
_____
_____
_____
_____
_____
_____
_____
_____
_____
_____

Day 19

Gone with the Wind...

I know that you've asked yourself for forgiveness. It's time to release those burdens. Use today to skim though your home for unwanted or useless items. Go from room to room – looking in the closets, basement, garage, or any other areas in the home that stores painful memories. Gather the items and prepare to get rid of them!

This is your day *for spring cleaning!*

I don't care how big or small the items are – just make sure you pack them up!!

They say, *'one man's trash can be another man's treasure'*. So use this opportunity to bless someone by donating your belongings to a shelter, non-profit org, or family in need. I don't care; just get rid of it.

Put a heart on this page when completed.

This exercise is symbolic to getting rid of things we know no longer serves us!

MY SUPPORTERS

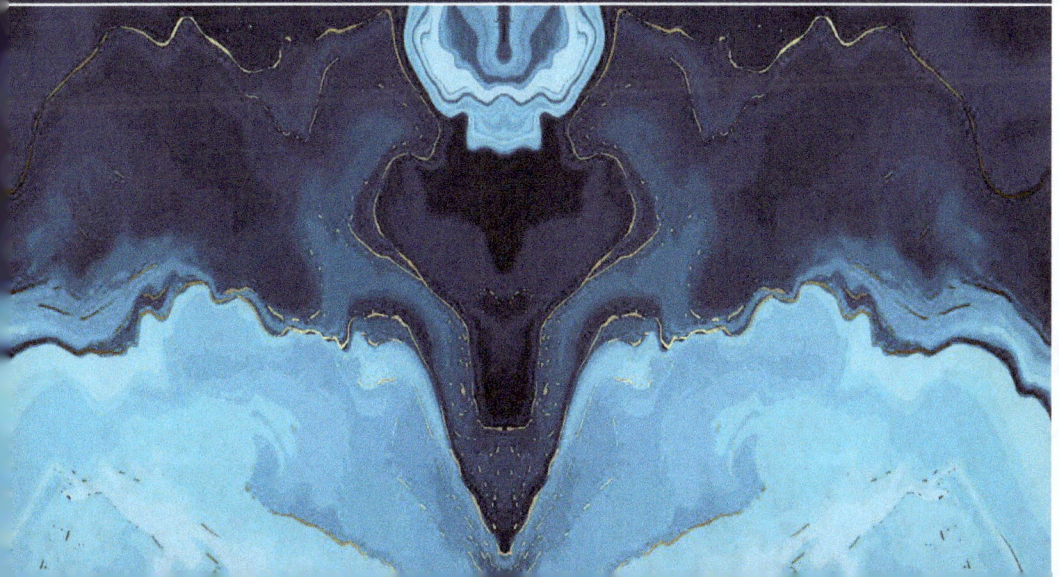

Day 20

Your 'One'

Most of the time, it's hard to see through those blurred lines. It took my best friend to tell me that I was making her feel "not enough"; even with what she was going through, she was still trying to be there for me. But when you're in YOUR SHIT, it's hard to care about, think about, sympathize with, or even acknowledge a person's presence, care, and effort to helping you get through.

Take this time to identify one person that has been present for you in your journey. Maybe identify someone who *tried* to be present and thank them for their efforts, love, and support. If no one comes to mind, write a letter to the person you'd *like* to be present and tell them how you'd want their love and support to look in this time for you.

Thank you Socks, this day is dedicated to YOU! 🤗

Letter to 'My One'

Day 21

Be ya Own Hype Man

So often we beat ourselves up for the choices we make, thoughts we have, people we love, the way we respond, the way we look, and so forth.

We are the most judgmental creation of God. Think about it – when potty-training dogs, people say 'discipline them in the moment or else seconds later they forget'! Animals don't live in future time; they are in the moment. They don't beat themselves up about not catching the meal of the day yesterday – they get back out, hunt, and move on. But we sit around and pity ourselves. We punish ourselves. And if the same or similar situation comes about again, we punish ourselves yet again as if the first time wasn't good enough. We have so much working against us that we forget to lift ourselves up. Forgiveness is key; praise is the lock.

Lock in those thoughts of all the amazing things that we overlook while punishing ourselves over and over and over.

Use this time to list 10 positive traits about yourself. Don't be humble! After you write out this list, go recite it in the mirror to YOURSELF.

Tear this page out and post it somewhere visible, so every morning when you look in the mirror you are reminded of the *WONDERFUL YOU*.

Ten Positive Traits

1. _____

2. _____

3. _____

4. _____

5. _____

6. _____

7. _____

8. _____

9. _____

10. _____

Day 22

The Village

Reality is – sometimes we become so depleted that we can't hold ourselves up. Carrying the burdens can sometimes seem daunting. You try to breathe but can't seem to catch your breath. We try to keep moving but seem stuck. We try to smile but end up crying. You try to stand up but you get knocked down. You try to take a step forward but it seems like you are constantly pushed backwards.

The solution to healing is COMMUNITY! No one is designed to go through the healing journey alone. We ALL need a village – whether it includes a therapist, family, friends, pastors, or whomever! A healthy journey requires "The Village".

Your village will consist of people that you trust, can be transparent with, will hold you accountable, and will lift you up during your dark days.

List up to 10 people that you call first when something major (whether good or bad) happens in your life. Explain why they are a part of your village.

My Village

Person 1: _____

Reason for Being in my Village: _____

_____

Person 2: _____

Reason for Being in my Village: _____

_____

Person 3: _____

Reason for Being in my Village: _____

_____

Person 4: _____

Reason for Being in my Village: _____

_____

Person 5: _____

Reason for Being in my Village: _____

_____

Person 6: _____

Reason for Being in my Village: _____

_____

Person 7: _____

Reason for Being in my Village: _____

_____

Person 8: _____

Reason for Being in my Village: _____

_____

Person 9: _____

Reason for Being in my Village: _____

_____

Person 10: _____

Reason for Being in my Village: _____

_____

Day 23

Rescue 911

Yes, we just discussed that people may not take the initiative to reach out and check on you. BUT that doesn't mean you don't need a village. Healing requires SUPPORT! One thing that I noticed while on this healing journey is that when you are deep in your shit – sometimes you can't articulate what you need and/or how you feel. What's even more frustrating is not being able to explain *why* you feel the way you feel. Not being able to identify where the feeling came from or what will help you feel better can be tormenting.

You give off the vibes of "leave me alone" when you really want a hug or someone to just sit with you without saying anything.

The saying *"closed mouths don't get fed"* is even true in the mental health realm. Most times, what we really need isn't projected through our actions. And that's mainly because we're confused about our emotions in those states. When emotions run high our clarity tends to be low.

Because of this, I've learned to teach people
how to love me when I'm down. I talk about certain activities that will get me moving, foods that cheer me up, what gestures or words to use that will produce a positive response in my brain.

For some family and friends, we've created code words to help them identify when I'm in a state of emotional need.

I hated feeling misunderstood, so a simple, *"I can tell you're not feeling well today, let's go for a walk"* would typically be a good pick-me-up for physical activity. Walking released hormones that made the load a little lighter and created the space for dialogue so I could vent and just get some things off my mind.

Who is a person you can call that is good for helping pull you out of that dark place? What hobbies can you do to keep you from sinking? (You may have already shared some of these on Day 0 or updated it on Day 16 this journal.)

Now is the time to be accountable and transparent. You being the only one who knows what helps you in times of despair does you no good. So review that list of people and be prepared to share these tools with someone you trust! When you call with that magical code word or complete silence, they will recognize this as your cry for help and will now know exactly what you need to feel better! Remember, it's best to be *proactive* rather than *reactive*.

Use this time to fill out our ESP ([Emotional Support Plan](#)) and share it with at least two people that you trust will be available when you are feeling low. It can be two people from your **Village**.

Emotional Support Plan (ESP)

Name: _____

· How will someone know that you're in a good mood?

· What are things you do to make yourself feel good? (hobbies, activities, etc.)

· What are your triggers/early warning signs that you aren't feeling well?

· What helps you feel better?

· What makes you feel worse?

List three people you can call when you're not feeling well.

_____

_____

_____

Community Resources:

_____

_____

_____

National Suicide Prevention Lifeline 1-800-273-8255

Samsha's National Helpline 1-800-662-HELP (4357)

Emotional Support Plan (ESP)

Name: _____

- How will someone know that you're in a good mood?

- What are things you do to make yourself feel good? (hobbies, activities, etc.)

- What are your triggers/early warning signs that you aren't feeling well?

- What helps you feel better?

- What makes you feel worse?

List three people you can call when you're not feeling well.

_____

_____

_____

Community Resources:

_____

_____

_____

National Suicide Prevention Lifeline 1-800-273-8255

Samsha's National Helpline 1-800-662-HELP (4357)

Day 24

Giving Back

We get so needy that we forget to appreciate those walking and crying with us. We subconsciously disregard those voices of reason in our lives.

The ones closest to us are the ones that we hurt the most. Truth of the matter is: no one is obligated to be here with or for us! Since we have identified our number one supporter and our village – now is the time to *show appreciation*.

Write a short letter of appreciation to both your number one and those listed as a part of your village. It's not mandatory to *deliver* the letters, but keep in mind everyone wants to feel appreciated – so I highly suggest you consider delivering them, if possible.

Letter of Appreciation

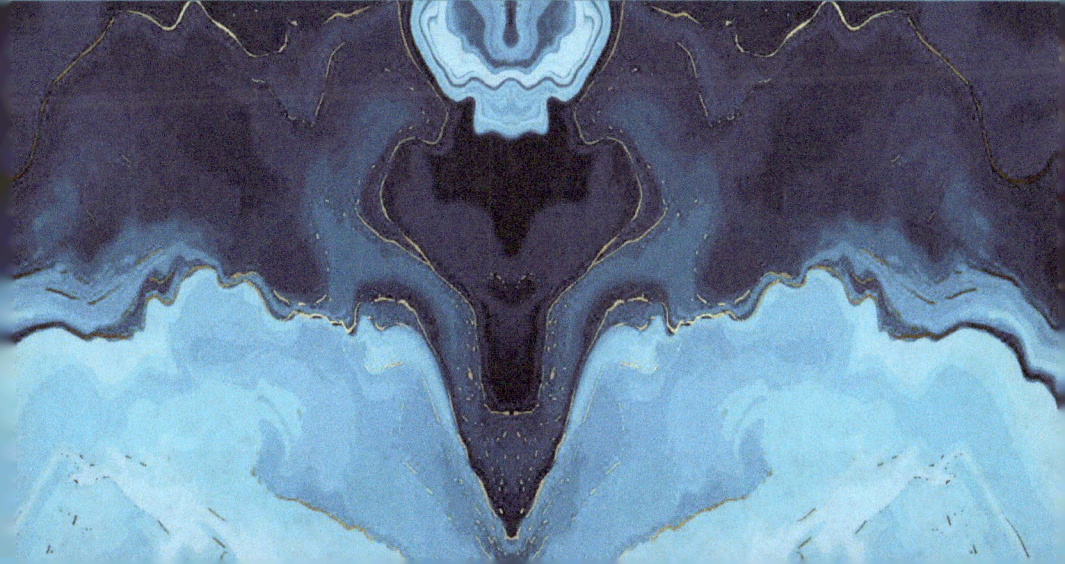

SELF CARE

Day 25

Day of Self-Care

Today is a day for YOU!

Love on YOU!

GRATITUDE JOURNAL

Date: _____   S M T W T F S

TODAY I'M GRATEFUL FOR

_____

_____

_____

TODAY'S AFFIRMATION

_____

_____

_____

SOMETHING I'M PROUD OF

_____

_____

_____

TOMORROW I LOOK FORWARD TO

_____

_____

_____

Feelings Grid

Intensity of Feelings	HAPPY	SAD	ANGRY	CONFUSED
High	Elated Excited Overjoyed Thrilled Exuberant Ecstatic Fired Up Delighted	Depressed Heartbroken Alone Hurt Unwanted Dejected Hopeless Sorrowful Crushed	Furious Enraged Outraged Aggravated Irate Seething	Bewildered Trapped Troubled Desperate Lost
Medium	Cheerful Up Good Relieved Satisfied Pleased	Disappointed Down Upset Distressed Regret Left Out	Upset Mad Annoyed Frustrated Agitated Hot Disgusted	Disorganized Foggy Misplaced Disoriented Mixed Up Lost
Low	Glad Satisfied Pleasant Fine Mellow	Unhappy Moody Blue Sorry Bad Dissatisfied	Perturbed Uptight Dismayed Irritated Discontent	Unsure Puzzled Bothered Uncomfortable Undecided Baffled Perplexed

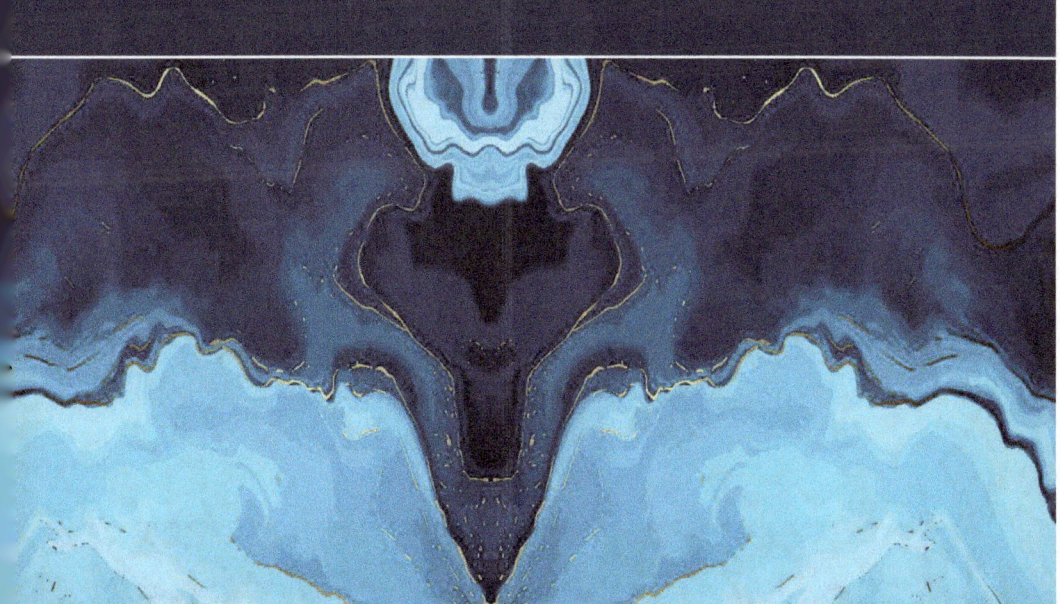

THE COME UP

Day 26

Joy Comes in the Morning

I'ma use this day to encourage you! Yes, this shit *sucks!* It hurts.

It's hard to see the light when you're in such a dark place but baby, let me tell you...all those cheesy cliches are TRUE!

What doesn't kill you makes you stronger.

Weeping may endure for a night, but joy comes in the morning. **(Psalm 30:5)**

There's light at the end of the tunnel...

These sayings are all true but it takes work to get there. And YOU can DO IT! I did it! It was hard as hell but there is a reward in *pressing through!!*

Most times when we are in our dark place, we can't think of anything outside of this current situation. It's hard to find joy. It's even harder trying to be positive when everything around you seems so dang ole *negative*. Well, I encourage you to shut all that negativity down just for today; JUST FOR THIS MOMENT!

It's okay to dream. Hell, if your journey is anything like mine – most dreams have become nightmares...so I dreaded going to sleep. I used my days to try and be as positive and optimistic as possible. Now I wasn't always successful at this task because – let's just keep it real – it's easy to sink in the funk! We are good at throwing pity parties baby, but today *let's celebrate life*! Because as hurtful as the reality is, some people didn't make it to this stage. Some people aren't alive to tell their story! Some weren't strong enough to push through and even though they may be alive, they aren't *living!*

So here's to TODAY! Here's to a second or maybe a third chance! We should all just be thankful for another chance and opportunity to *get it right!*

Challenge yourself to think BIG!

Write down things that make you happy, things that you desire to do in the very near future, and things on your bucket list. I don't care if it's traveling, starting a company, or writing a book/journal 😊. Just write! All positivity! Write about things that are attainable within the next day, month, years, or even *decades.* JUST WRITE!

Now go back and circle one thing that you can commit to doing over *the next week!* Just circle it and let life have its way!

Day 27

What's to Come

The changes I'm going through…I'll never be the same…

How does one bounce back from pain?

How does one survive heartache without impacting the next relationship or friendship?

HEAL!!

But what exactly *is* healing? Everyone has their own methods of healing, so I'd say there's no incorrect answer. Do what makes you feel good.

A lot of people tried to get me to sit still as part of my healing. And honestly, this has been the first time I've actually done just that – sat STILL!

Sat in my thoughts and my pain. Processed my trauma. Asked myself many questions, answered many questions. But at the end of the day, my healing comes from helping others process through the same pain I've endured. Do I purposely put myself through things just to say I've been through it? No! But I do take advantage of my experiences and use my voice to help others – because that's my calling! God gave me a voice, personality, and heart to be who I am. Resiliency is in me and it keeps me going. It keeps me fighting and pushing through. And it wasn't until *THIS TRAUMA* that I realized how strong I really was!

Every day something happened that reminded me of the pain, trauma, and consequences I had to endure behind another's actions. Yet every day I cried – I got up and tackled each challenge with confidence that *if I get through this I'll make it to the finish line*. I wanted to see the blessings waiting for me…so I pressed though.

I often asked would I love or trust the same. And the answer was *no!* No lessons learned should produce the same results. You go through things; you learn and you grow.

So, I promised to *grow* from this. This pain changed me.

I'll always be a lover. I love love! I love feeling love and I love loving. But what I learned in this experience is realizing what makes me feel loved and ensuring it doesn't stem from trauma. Understanding what true, unconditional love is and promising to give that to myself FIRST! That way someone else's love is a bonus and NOT mandatory!

Love shouldn't be forced. When it's forced, it essentially becomes a piece that won't *fit* and at some point the whole puzzle will fall apart! Learning that *'I'm ENOUGH'* was the hardest part of my journey. But *me being worth it* doesn't equate to being enough to fight for. It's knowing *who I am and what I bring to the table* **is** *good enough for one person to honor.* Knowing that my flaws will be looked at and prayed over with patience and care to accompany the journey.

Use this time to journal about how you can use your passion for the good in the future.

Day 28

Grateful

When I sit back and reflect on all the obstacles I've overcome – I feel blessed! Reflecting on all of the people and things that tore me down, were sent to destroy me, and intended to block my path – I realize that here I am today, still standing prosperous in one piece!

I can't help but to believe that *there is a God!*

Write a letter of gratitude to the power in which you believe in!

Letter of Gratitude

Day 29

You Got the Pen

One the most frustrating parts of this journey was *ignoring the rumors*. Everybody speculated. I had people randomly sending friend requests, inquiring on why I was no longer wearing my wedding ring! Seriously, they were even commenting on pictures! Smh! When I decided to move on and start dating, people swore I was still married because I never announced my divorce. Even to this day, I'm positive there are a few people reading this journal and finally getting my side once and for all. I knew that in order to heal from this, I had to keep quiet until I was emotionally ready for people to really hear MY STORY – from ME!

Everybody tries to write your story and tell your business. Take the pen back and tell it in your own words!

Take this time to *write your autobiography!*

If the only thing people knew about you was what they read on this page, what do you want the world to remember about you?

#InspireOne

Autobiography

_____
_____
_____
_____
_____
_____
_____
_____
_____
_____
_____
_____
_____
_____
_____
_____
_____
_____
_____
_____
_____
_____
_____
_____
_____

Day 30

End of Book

Wow! Congratulations! You've made it to the end of your 30-day healing process.

As life happens, it's hard to stop and deal with the current pains. But it's so necessary to **sit in your shit!** It helps process and prioritize, but more so it helps with analyzing and redirecting! It allows us to hold ourselves accountable to focusing on us while dealing with our real and raw emotions – and YOU DID THAT!

I'm so proud of you!

I promise this was the hardest, yet most rewarding process for me to take when I was going through my second divorce! And it was EVERYTHING. I didn't know that I needed to but I'm glad I did it. So, I can relate to where you are and from me to you – I want to be the first to say I'M PROUD OF YOU! BE PROUD OF YOURSELF!

Being intentional is never easy! But you did it!

Being uncomfortable is – *by definition* – never comfortable, but you pushed through!

Again, I'm so proud of you! Fortunately, you've done the hard part! You sat in that shit and you dealt with the hurt, confusion, and maybe even some happy thoughts that came about!

Now the next step is to *commit to continuing the process!*

I'd like to offer you a gift for your bravery! As a life coach, I'd like to offer you a discounted rate to book our 6-week package to continue your healing journey.

Life coaching is not the same as therapy as it doesn't include a medical diagnosis. However, life coaching is having access to a trained and knowledgeable adviser who will partner with you to provide ongoing support and guidance as you continue to reach your potential. Everything you discuss with your coach is confidential, so you can speak freely without judgement.

Together, we can create an action plan to move you towards your goals and help you to achieve your desired future.

The 6-week program includes six (6) weekly 45-minute sessions at a 50% discount for you choosing to complete this journal!

Visit our website now to sign up for this package using the promo code GIFT and let's get ready to further your journey of HEALING!

See ya soon,

— *Devin Elisse*

Additional Journaling Pages

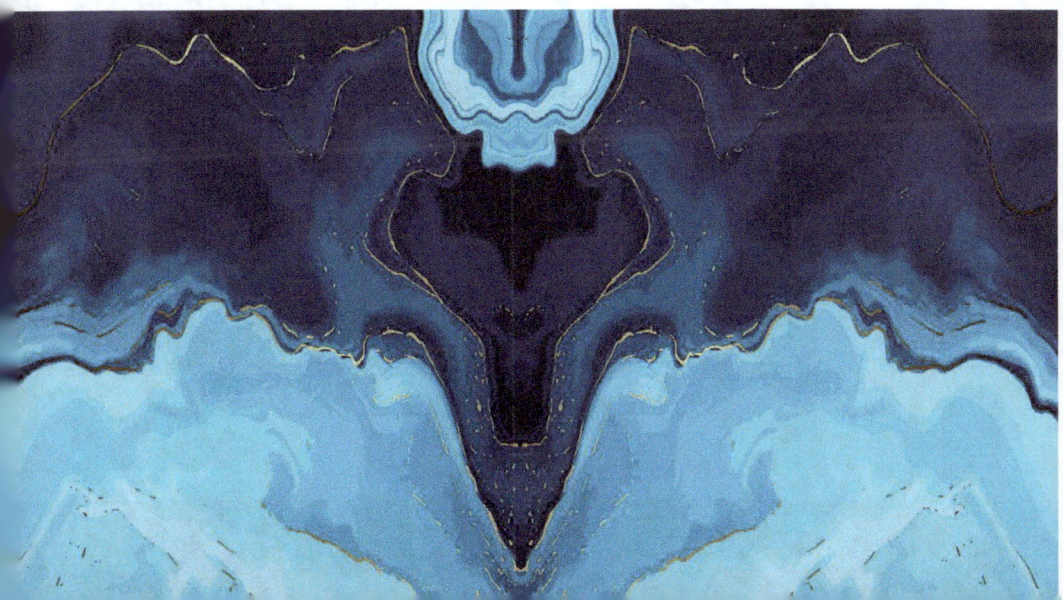

ABOUT THE AUTHOR

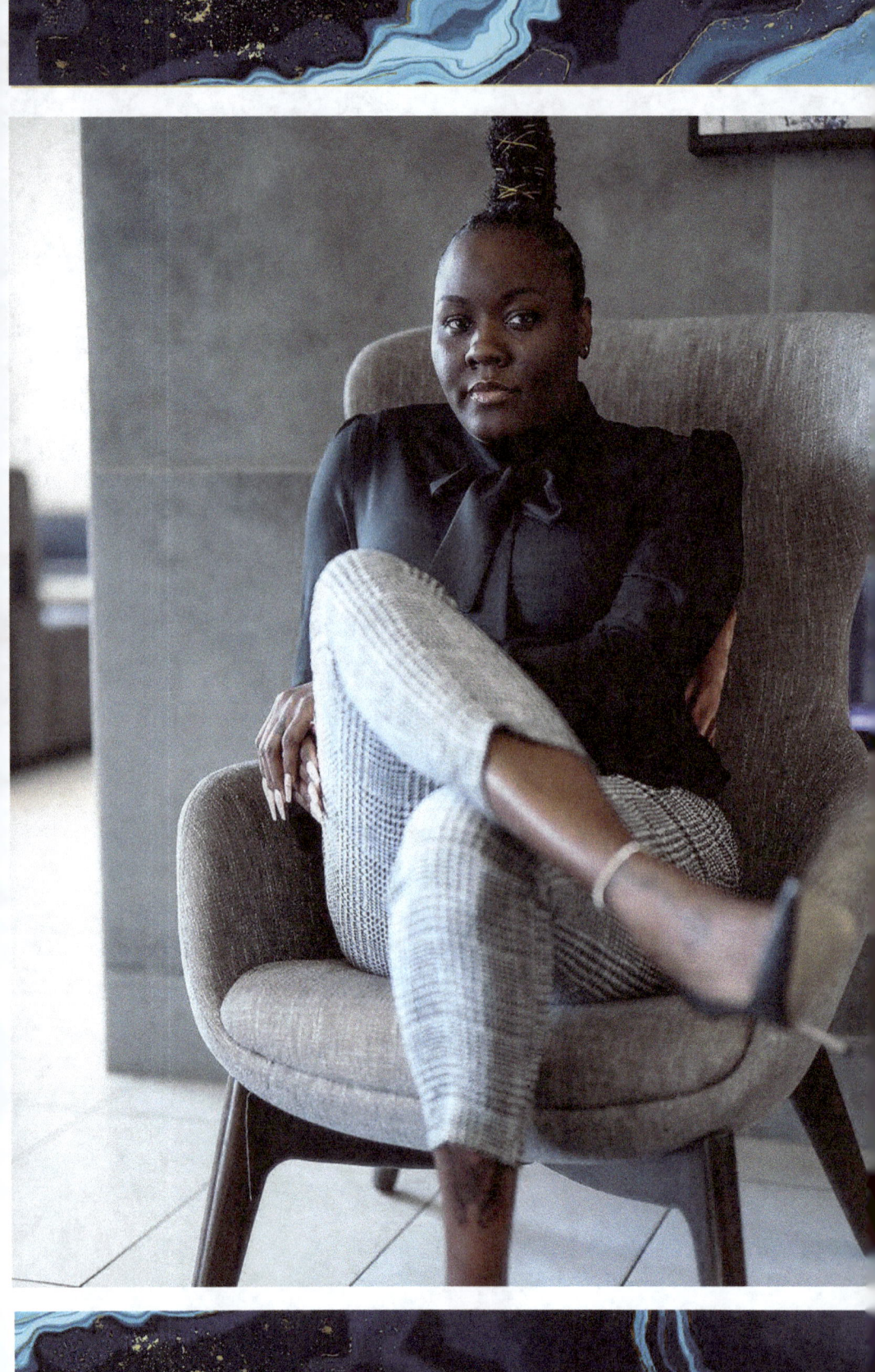

Devin Elisse

Devin Elisse is the founder of **Lifted KC**, a local mental health nonprofit in Kansas City, MO that was originally started after Devin faced personal struggles with postpartum depression. Learning to understand her condition and not accept simply being labeled as "different" to the world created this ever-growing passion for addressing trauma and healing.

Evolving into a published author, Devin now seeks to help guide people along their healing journey through written works. Devin believes her experience with healing from her own childhood and adult traumas has opened the door to her newfound calling, "serving and advocating for the mental health community."

Devin received certification from the State of Missouri as a Peer Specialist where she uses that license to coach those directly affected with mental health struggles. She received certifications in *Mental Health First Aid* for both *Youth* and *Adults*, and later became a facilitator for the *Mental Health First Aid Youth* curriculum. Devin currently partners with **NAMI** to coordinate their *"Ending the Silence"* presentation. She also provides training classes to those seeking to be a support in the mental health community.

Her first written work, ***"Sit In Yo Shit"*** is published under *EMEYEU Literature* and *Truth's Haven*, the empowerment & non-fiction imprints of the black-owned publishing company.

Contact Devin Elisse

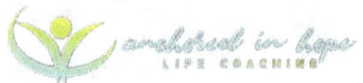

Devin Elisse is a certified life coach through her company, Anchored in Hope, which serves individuals who are ready to transform their lives and center hope into their journey.

Contact Devin:

www.anchorednhope.org

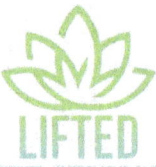

anchoredkc@gmail.com

Founded by Devin Elisse, this organization seeks to reduce the stigma associated with mental health by promoting awareness of mental illness, its symptoms, and providing resources for those in need.

www.liftedkc.org

liftedkcorg@gmail.com

Contact Devin Elisse (cont.)

Follow on Facebook and Instagram: @liftedkc_org

Also Follow Devin Elisse

on

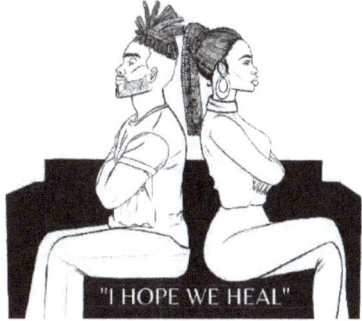

The featured podcast from Angela Marie Publishing centered around mental health in the Black Community.

Listen on Spotify or YouTube:

Follow on Facebook: @theBlackedOutCouch

www.ingramcontent.com/pod-product-compliance
Lightning Source LLC
Chambersburg PA
CBHW071325120626
46546CB00002B/450

www.ingramcontent.com/pod-product-compliance
Lightning Source LLC
Chambersburg PA
CBHW061138120626
46546CB00005B/1844